AF882407

It's easy to get lost in the cancer world

Let NCCN Guidelines for Patients® be your guide

- ✓ Step-by-step guides to the cancer care options likely to have the best results
- ✓ Based on treatment guidelines used by health care providers worldwide
- ✓ Designed to help you discuss cancer treatment with your doctors

National Comprehensive Cancer Network®

NCCN Guidelines for Patients® are developed by the National Comprehensive Cancer Network® (NCCN®)

NCCN

- An alliance of leading cancer centers across the United States devoted to patient care, research, and education

Cancer centers that are part of NCCN:
NCCN.org/cancercenters

NCCN Clinical Practice Guidelines in Oncology (NCCN Guidelines®)

- Developed by experts from NCCN cancer centers using the latest research and years of experience
- For providers of cancer care all over the world
- Expert recommendations for cancer screening, diagnosis, and treatment

Free online at
NCCN.org/guidelines

NCCN Guidelines for Patients

- Present information from the NCCN Guidelines in an easy-to-learn format
- For people with cancer and those who support them
- Explain the cancer care options likely to have the best results

Free online at
NCCN.org/patientguidelines

These NCCN Guidelines for Patients are based on the NCCN Guidelines® for Antiemesis, Version 2.2022 — March 23, 2022.

© 2022 National Comprehensive Cancer Network, Inc. All rights reserved. NCCN Guidelines for Patients and illustrations herein may not be reproduced in any form for any purpose without the express written permission of NCCN. No one, including doctors or patients, may use the NCCN Guidelines for Patients for any commercial purpose and may not claim, represent, or imply that the NCCN Guidelines for Patients that have been modified in any manner are derived from, based on, related to, or arise out of the NCCN Guidelines for Patients. The NCCN Guidelines are a work in progress that may be redefined as often as new significant data become available. NCCN makes no warranties of any kind whatsoever regarding its content, use, or application and disclaims any responsibility for its application or use in any way.

NCCN Foundation seeks to support the millions of patients and their families affected by a cancer diagnosis by funding and distributing NCCN Guidelines for Patients. NCCN Foundation is also committed to advancing cancer treatment by funding the nation's promising doctors at the center of innovation in cancer research. For more details and the full library of patient and caregiver resources, visit NCCN.org/patients.

National Comprehensive Cancer Network (NCCN) / NCCN Foundation
3025 Chemical Road, Suite 100
Plymouth Meeting, PA 19462
215.690.0300

NCCN Guidelines for Patients are supported by funding from the NCCN Foundation®

To make a gift or learn more, please visit NCCNFoundation.org/donate
or e-mail PatientGuidelines@NCCN.org.

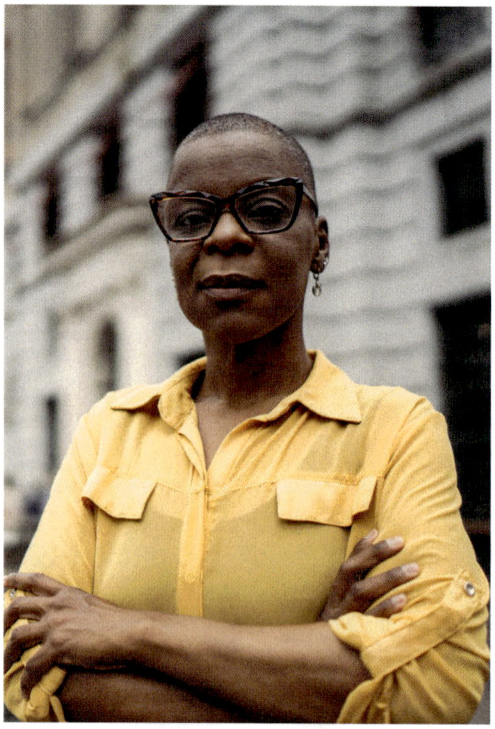
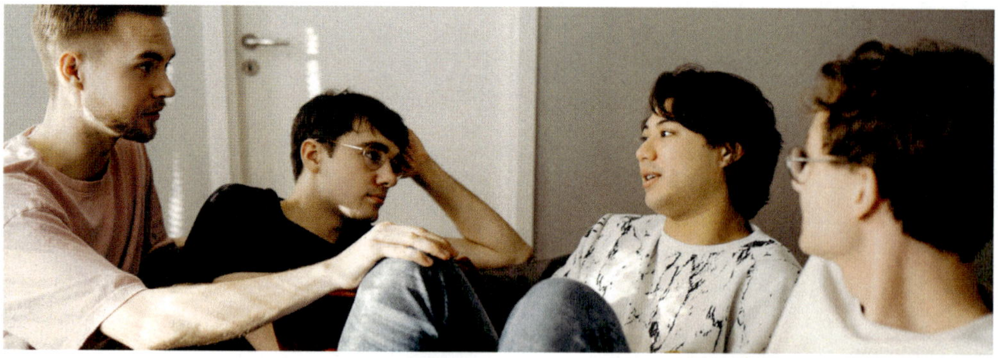
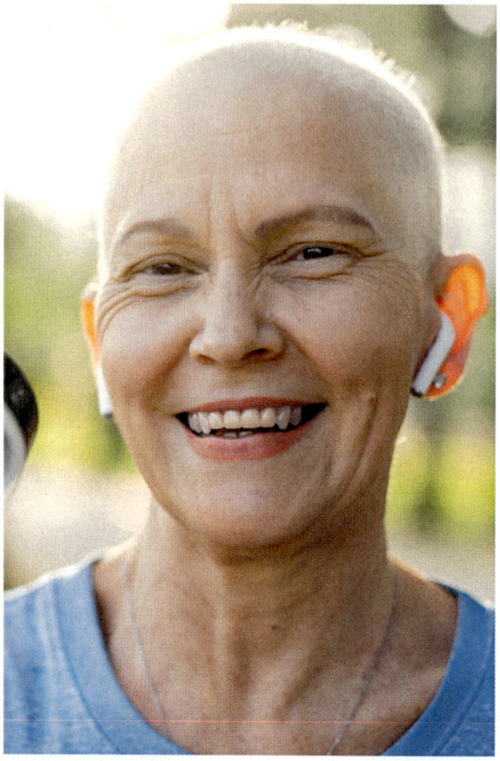
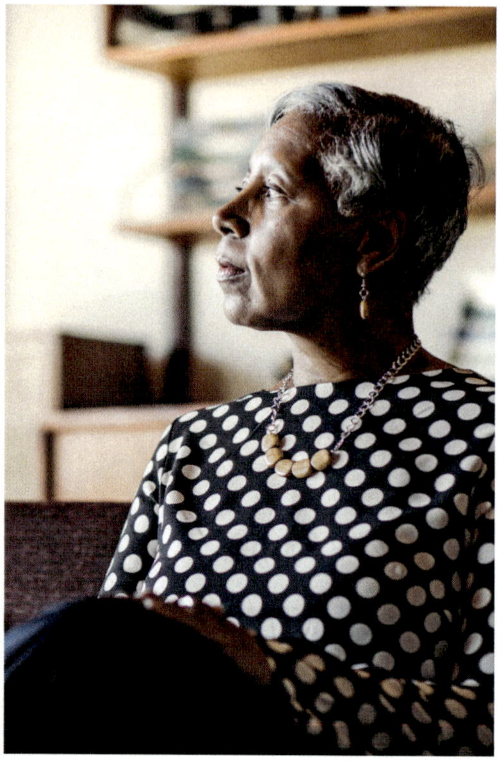
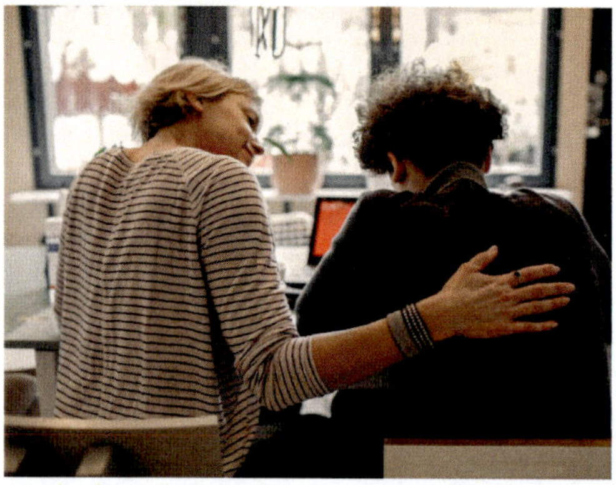
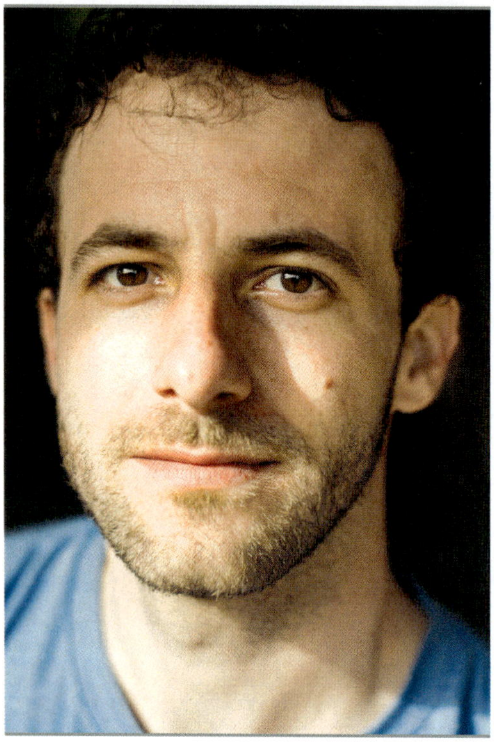
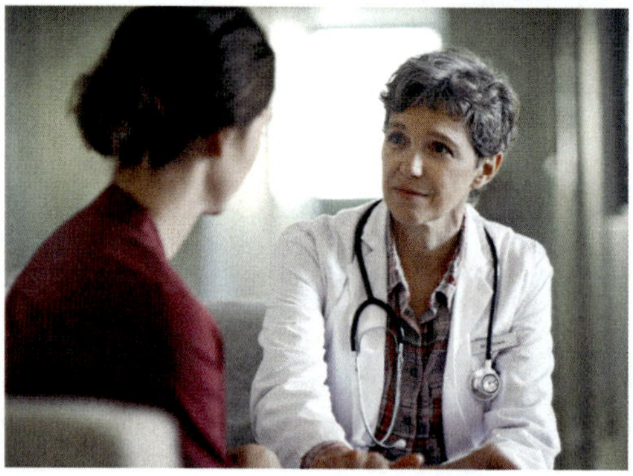
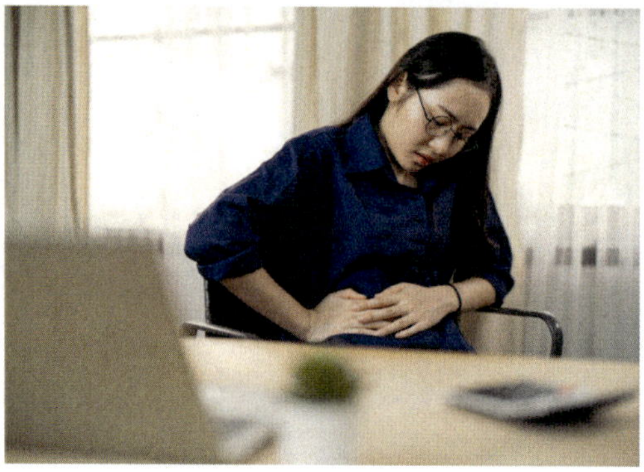
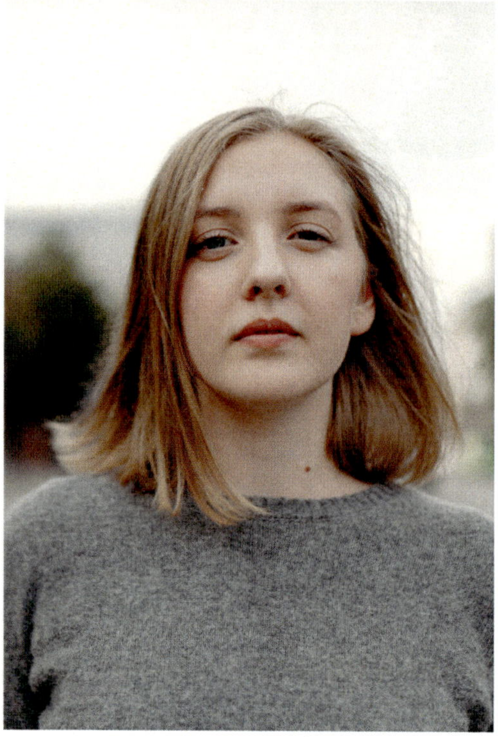

Contents

1 Nausea and vomiting basics

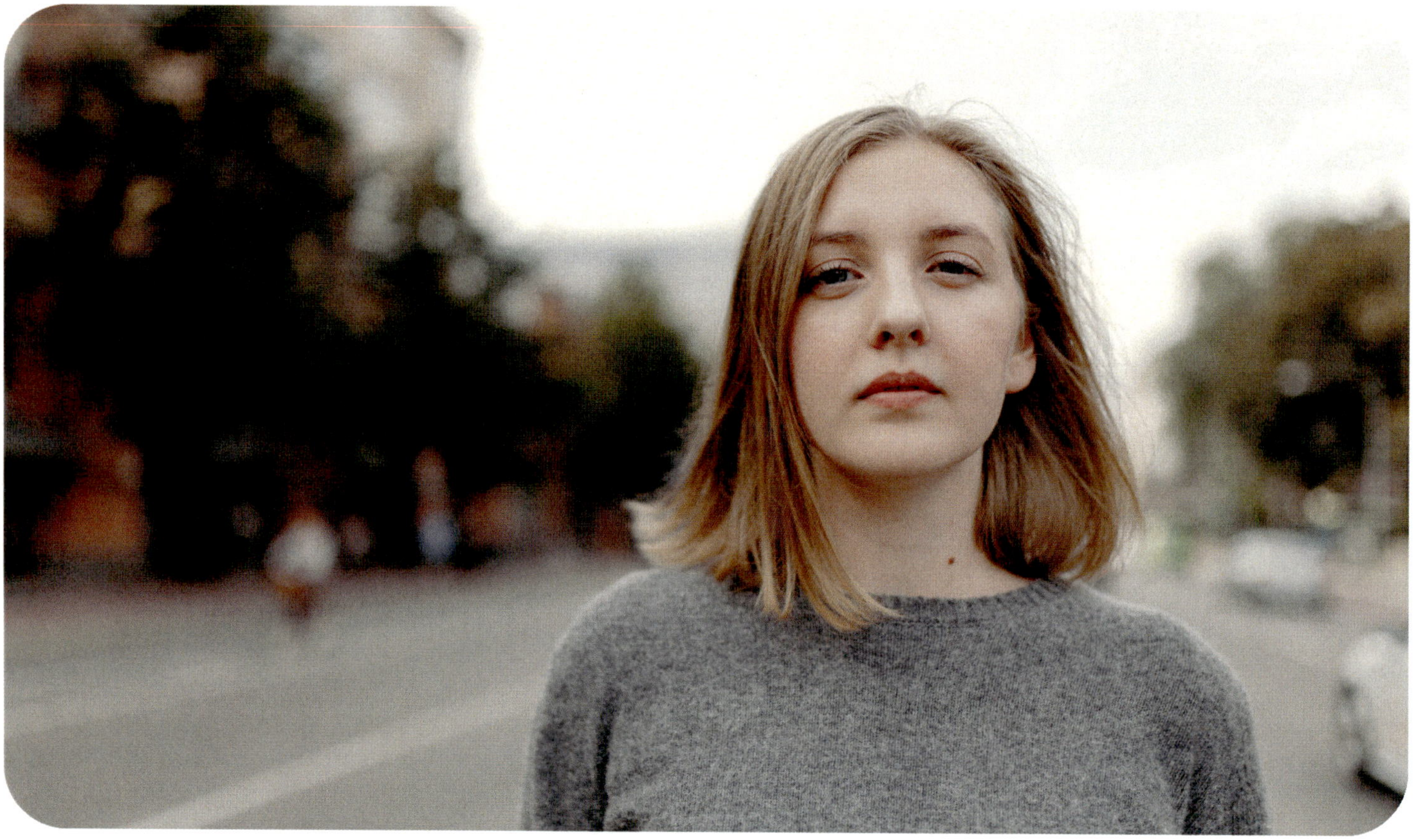

Nausea and vomiting are common but often preventable side effects of cancer treatment. In other words, your life doesn't have to come to a complete stop because you're receiving cancer medications. This chapter explains the basics of nausea and vomiting, and what you can do about these side effects.

Having cancer and undergoing cancer treatment can be very stressful. You may feel a wide range of emotions and discomforts. Your care team wants to help you focus on your treatment. But sometimes the side effects caused by cancer treatment can overshadow the treatment itself.

Nausea and vomiting are two side effects of cancer treatment that patients often fear.

- **Nausea** is that sensation when you feel like you're going to throw up. You feel woozy, queasy, or sick to your stomach. Nausea often comes before vomiting but it can also occur without vomiting.
- **Vomiting** is forcefully throwing up what's in your stomach. It usually comes out of your mouth but can also come out through your nose. Frequent vomiting can affect your quality of life, your overall well-being, and may lead to dehydration.

Not every patient gets sick from cancer therapy. But if you have these side effects, it's important to reduce them as much as possible to prevent them from interfering with your treatment.

What causes nausea and vomiting?

Nausea and vomiting are reflexes that happen when your body wants to get rid of harmful (toxic) substances in the intestine and stomach. Nausea and vomiting can occur together or separately.

This book is about nausea and vomiting that comes from cancer treatments like chemotherapy and radiation therapy. This book also explains what you need to know about preventing nausea and vomiting.

Medications used to prevent and treat nausea and vomiting have come a long way over the years. Today, nausea and vomiting can be managed and even prevented. When they can't be prevented, there are other ways to help you cope.

How are nausea and vomiting prevented?

Your doctors and care team will develop a treatment plan just for you that will help reduce or prevent these side effects.

Prevention is the key. It's important to try to prevent these side effects before they develop. It's easier to prevent them than treat them—after nausea and vomiting start, they're much harder to stop.

This plan will also help you cope if prevention doesn't work or comes too late.

- *Emesis* is the medical term for vomiting.
- *Antiemesis* is the term for preventing nausea and vomiting.
- *Antiemetics* are medications for preventing or relieving nausea and vomiting.

The first step is for your doctors and care team to learn all they can about you. This includes specifics about you as well as your medical history of nausea and vomiting.

Other things your care team will consider when planning how to prevent nausea and vomiting are listed in Guide 1.

What can nausea and vomiting do to your body?

Nausea and vomiting can be serious and cause harm to your body, especially if they happen repeatedly. Nausea and vomiting that aren't treated can get worse with time. Nausea and vomiting can also interrupt or delay your treatment schedule.

Nausea and vomiting can cause you to:

- Not want to eat
- Lose fluids (become dehydrated)
- Be low in electrolytes, which are minerals that your body needs to function

Guide 1
Things to consider when making an antiemesis plan

Cancer treatment information:
• The type of treatment you'll get
• How much of the treatment you'll get (dose)
• When and how often you'll get the treatment
• Whether the treatment is a pill, an IV, or other
Risk factors:
• Age
• Sex (male or female)
• Past cancer treatments
• History of drinking alcohol
• Motion sickness
• History of morning sickness (during pregnancy)
• Feelings of anxiety
• Current medications

- Miss out on vitamins you need from food or drink
- Lose the energy you need to carry out your daily activities
- Reduce your body's ability to heal wounds
- Possibly cause tearing of your esophagus (the tube-shaped organ between your throat and stomach)
- Alter your ability to function normally in your mind and body
- Cancel or delay necessary cancer treatment

Nausea can come on within hours after treatment (acute) or it can take a day or more (delayed). When nausea is delayed, it can be more intense and harder to treat. You can become dehydrated and need fluids, which are given through an IV (intravenous) tube inserted into your body.

When are antiemetics needed?

When patients feel sick, they may cancel or postpone their cancer treatment. Your doctors don't want anything to stop or delay your treatment. Delaying your treatment may prolong or cause difficulties with your cancer.

The goal is to prevent you from feeling sick in the first place. You want to stay ahead of the symptoms.

Depending on your cancer treatment, you may need to use a combination of antiemetic medications. These medications work best if taken on a schedule or as soon as you begin to feel a little queasy.

Stick to the schedule and the instructions you received with your antiemetic drugs. Make sure you use these medications at the right times and at the correct dosage. Don't skip a scheduled dose even if you feel fine. If you wait until you start feeling sick, it may be too late for the medication to work.

Can I ask for antiemetics?

If your doctor or care team hasn't already talked to you about anti-nausea and antiemetic drugs, you should certainly ask about them.

Many experts believe that anti-nausea and anti-vomiting medications aren't used as often as they should be. This is a problem that involves both patients and health care providers. Some patients feel that they don't want to bother their care team with questions. Or they've heard that cancer treatment is *supposed to* cause nausea and vomiting—that these side effects are a routine part of treatment.

Preventing nausea and vomiting is the goal. Once these side effects start, they can be difficult to stop.

At the same time, some care providers may underestimate how often nausea and vomiting occur or how disruptive these side effects can be for patients.

If your doctor or care team isn't aware you're feeling sick, they may not ask you about it. But they do want to help. So if you develop any side effects from your cancer treatment, don't try to "tough it out." Call your care team and let them know right away, whether it's day or night.

Also, if you've been given anti-nausea or antiemetic medications but they're not working or you don't like their side effects, let your care team know about that, too. There are a lot of options to treat nausea and vomiting.

share with us.

Take our survey
and help make the NCCN Guidelines for Patients better for everyone!

NCCN.org/patients/comments

Nausea can develop within hours after cancer treatment (acute) or it can take one or more days to develop (delayed). Delayed nausea is a common result of cancer treatment.

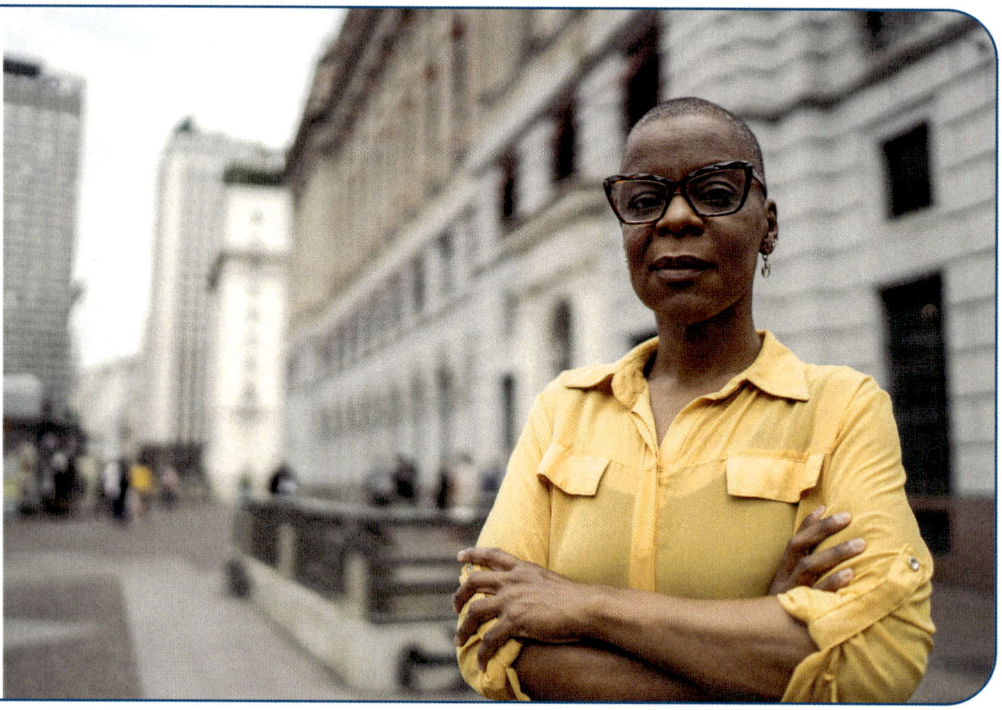

Key points

- Nausea is the feeling that you are going to throw up.
- Vomiting (emesis) is forcefully throwing up what's in your stomach.
- Antiemesis means preventing or stopping nausea and vomiting. An antiemetic is a drug that prevents or lessens nausea and vomiting.
- Preventing nausea and vomiting is the goal. Once these side effects start, it's much harder to stop them.
- Nausea can come on within hours after treatment (acute) or within days after treatment (delayed).
- Nausea and vomiting can cause harm to your body, especially if they happen repeatedly.
- Don't skip a scheduled dose of antiemetic medication, even if you're feeling fine.
- Delaying your treatment may prolong or cause difficulties with your cancer.

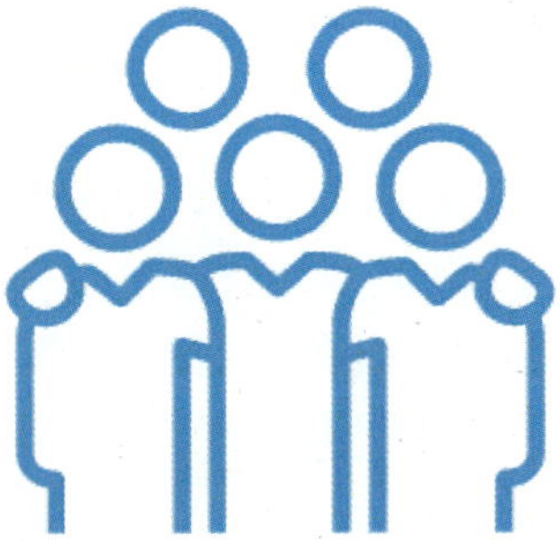

When to contact your care team

Nausea and vomiting can be caused by medical conditions unrelated to your cancer treatment. It's important to call your care team if:

- You continue to have nausea and vomiting from cancer treatment despite taking antiemetics.
- Nausea interferes with your ability to eat.
- Vomiting occurs 4 to 5 times in a 24-hour period.
- You feel bloated.
- You have pain or a swollen stomach before nausea and vomiting occurs.
- You're bothered by the side effects from your antiemetic medications.

What happens when you vomit?

Vomiting is when the stomach forcefully empties what's inside, which comes out of the mouth as vomit. It's the body's way of protecting itself from harmful substances or germs.

But how exactly does it happen? Here's a simplified step-by-step description.

Step 1

A harmful substance (such as germs, alcohol, or a chemotherapy drug) enters the body. Or a sensation (pain, anxiety, or motion) affects the body.

Step 2

Special receptors in different areas of the body (stomach, brain, ear, and more) detect the harmful substance or sensation.

Step 3

These receptors send danger signals to an area of the brain called the chemoreceptor trigger zone.

Step 4

The chemoreceptor trigger zone activates another mechanism in the brain called the vomiting center. (Some danger signals bypass the chemoreceptor trigger zone and go directly to the vomiting center.)

Step 5

The vomiting center jumps into action. It sends out a series of orders to several areas of the body to perform specific functions. It transmits signals to:

- The intestine and stomach, which contract and begin to shove the stomach contents upward.
- The vomiting center, which opens up a valve between the stomach and the esophagus (the tube-shaped organ between your throat and stomach) so that the vomit can continue upward.
- The diaphragm and the inner walls of the abdomen, which also contract.
- The lungs, which expand.

These actions close off the airway (to prevent vomit from entering it) and propel the vomit up the throat and out of the mouth.

Breaking the chain of events

Several key interactions happen throughout this sequence of events. This is when anti-nausea and anti-vomiting medications get to work. These medications block the signals at different points of communication between the stomach and the brain. This interrupts or shuts down a part of the sequence. Researchers still haven't developed a drug that will stop the entire vomiting process all at once (but they're working on it). That's why some people need 2 or more antiemetic medications to get relief.

2

Causes of nausea and vomiting

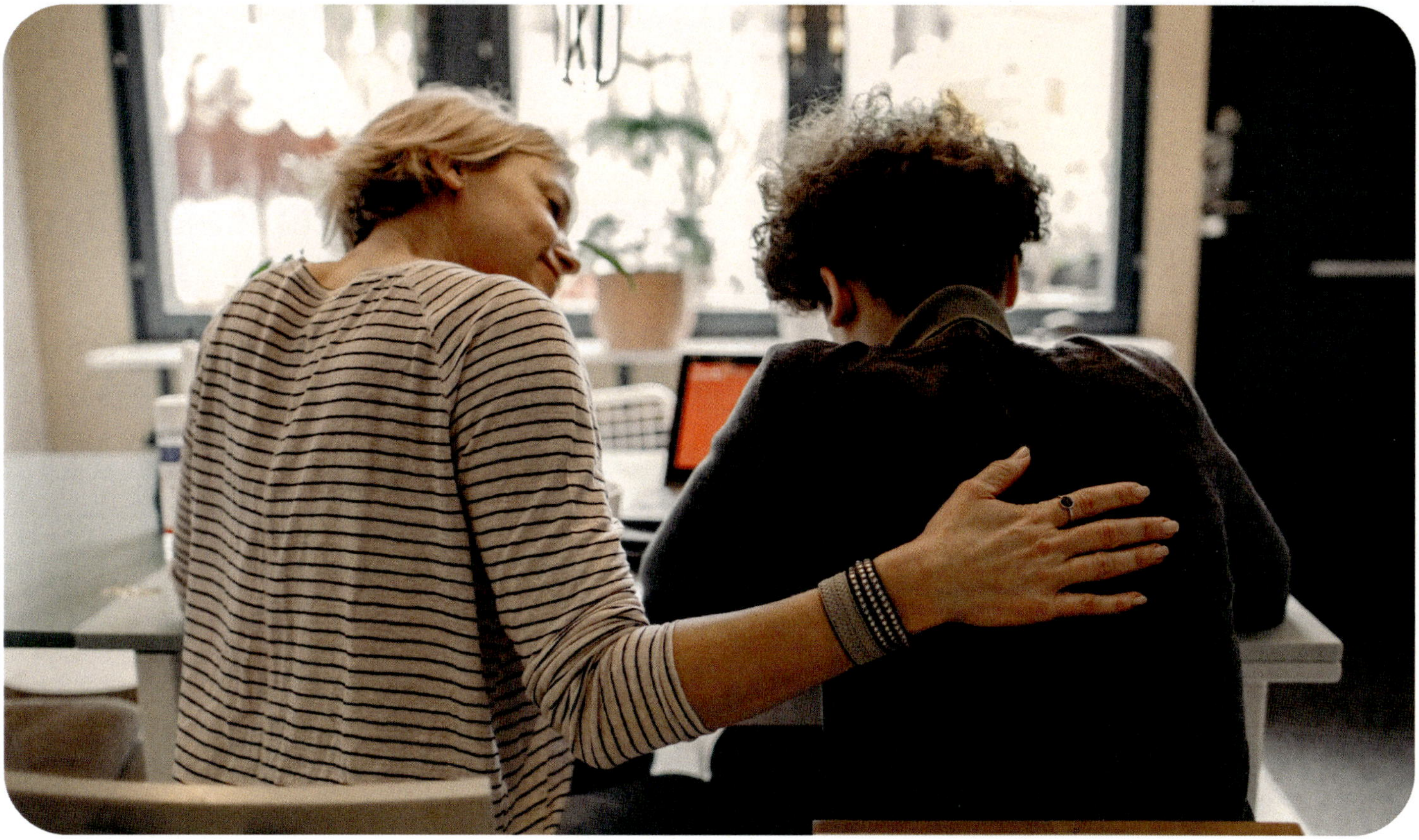

Many things can cause nausea and vomiting. This chapter explains which cancer treatments can cause these side effects. Nausea and vomiting can happen before, during, and after cancer treatment.

Nausea and vomiting are two of the most common side effects of cancer treatment. (Other side effects of cancer treatment include constipation, diarrhea, fatigue, hair loss, itchy skin, infections, mouth problems, and other effects. These aren't covered in this book.)

Side effects can happen from the cancer itself, from health problems caused by cancer, and from cancer treatment. Sometimes it can be difficult to tell the difference between the side effects of cancer treatment and the symptoms of the cancer itself.

> Every cancer therapy has a risk of causing side effects. These side effects can happen before, during, or after treatment.
>
> Sometimes cancer therapies are combined, which may increase the risk of side effects.

Other cancer-related causes of nausea and vomiting

Besides cancer therapy, other factors can cause nausea and vomiting in people with cancer. These include:

- Anxiety
- Infection
- Balance issues
- Cancer that spreads to the brain
- Lack of minerals in the body (electrolyte imbalance)
- Other drugs' side effects (for example, drugs for pain)
- Your intestine is blocked or you're very constipated
- Food staying in your stomach for too long
- Abnormal buildup of fluid in the belly area (abdomen)

Cancer treatments that cause nausea and vomiting

Many cancer treatments can cause nausea and vomiting:

- **Chemotherapy** uses drugs that disrupt rapidly dividing cells, including cancer cells and healthy cells. Chemotherapy is the most common cause of nausea and vomiting related to cancer treatment.
- **Radiation therapy** uses high-energy particles or rays to kill cancer cells. Radiation causes nausea and vomiting

when it affects rapidly dividing cells in the intestine.

- **Targeted therapy** seeks out and blocks how cancer cells grow and move in the body. Though targeted therapy can cause nausea and vomiting, it's more likely to cause other side effects.
- **Immunotherapy** boosts the body's immune system to find and destroy cancer cells. Immunotherapy can cause different side effects, some severe but most mild. One side effect is colitis, an inflammation of the colon. Symptoms of colitis include stomach cramps, diarrhea, bloody stools (poop), and nausea and vomiting.

The side effects you're likely to have depend on the type of cancer treatment you get. For example, chemotherapy can cause more side effects than other cancer therapies, such as targeted therapy and immunotherapy.

The amount (dose) of chemotherapy or radiation therapy can also have an effect on your body. Higher doses often cause more severe side effects. Your body can react to these therapies as if they're harmful or poisonous. Indeed, chemotherapy and radiation therapy are like poisons that attack and kill the cancer cells inside your body.

The nausea and vomiting related to chemotherapy, targeted therapy, and immunotherapy are grouped together and called chemotherapy-induced nausea and vomiting. The nausea and vomiting related to radiation is called radiation-induced nausea and vomiting. (The term "induced" means "to bring on something.")

Chemotherapy-induced nausea and vomiting

Chemotherapy is a systemic (whole-body) drug therapy that attacks fast-dividing cancer cells. It can also damage normal cells in the process. Damage to normal cells causes side effects. Targeted therapy and immunotherapy also cause side effects.

There are several different types of chemotherapy-induced nausea and vomiting. These types include acute, delayed, anticipatory, breakthrough, and refractory. Read about the different types of chemotherapy-induced nausea and vomiting in Guide 2.

A note about nausea

Although it seems like nausea and vomiting are two phases of the same illness, they may be separate conditions. Nausea often occurs without vomiting during cancer treatment or pregnancy, for example. Antiemetics can prevent or greatly reduce vomiting, but they may be less effective against nausea.

Guide 2
Types of chemotherapy-induced nausea and vomiting

Acute nausea and vomiting occur soon after cancer therapy (within minutes to hours).

- Acute nausea and vomiting usually stop within the first 24 hours of cancer therapy.
- The intensity hits its peak after 5 to 6 hours and then begins to lessen.
- Acute is linked to the type and amount of cancer treatment given, the environment where it's given, patient-specific factors (risk factors), and the patient's history of nausea and vomiting.

Delayed nausea and vomiting occur more than 24 hours after treatment is given.

- Delayed nausea is often more common, more severe, and more resistant to treatment than acute nausea.
- Delayed nausea and vomiting commonly occur with chemotherapy drugs that have a high risk of causing vomiting, such as cisplatin, carboplatin, cyclophosphamide, or doxorubicin.
- With cisplatin, vomiting can last for 6 to 7 days. Vomiting is at its worst about 2 to 3 days after cisplatin is given.

Anticipatory nausea and vomiting occur in anticipation of the next treatment to be given.

- Anticipatory nausea and vomiting come from an emotional or physical reaction to a past bad experience when getting treatment. (Anticipatory means expecting something to happen.) The patient anxiously expects the bad experience to happen again.
- Anticipatory nausea and vomiting can be triggered by smells, sights, or sounds related to treatment.
- Younger people with cancer are more likely to have this type.
- Younger people also may be more likely to develop this type because they have less control over vomiting.
- Nausea is more common than vomiting with this type. Anti-anxiety medication seems to help.

Breakthrough nausea and vomiting happen despite prevention with antiemetic drugs.

- Additional or different antiemetic drugs are used for breakthrough nausea and vomiting.

Refractory nausea and vomiting keep happening after each treatment cycle.

- Antiemetics haven't been able to control nausea or vomiting in previous treatment cycles. So nausea and vomiting keep coming back with each following cycle.
- Medication to prevent nausea or vomiting just isn't working.

Radiation-induced nausea and vomiting

Radiation therapy is a systemic therapy that often uses a large machine to transmit high-energy rays (radiation) to kill cancer cells. The risk of nausea and vomiting gets higher as the doses of radiation get larger and more frequent, and reach more areas of the body.

Radiation therapy aims to kill rapidly dividing cancer cells. The radiation may also damage healthy tissue, causing side effects. Radiation that treats the upper abdomen or whole body may reach the stomach and intestine (the long section of the digestive system that absorbs nutrients from food). Because the digestive system has many rapidly dividing cells, it's sensitive to radiation treatment. So when the stomach and the intestine receive radiation, nausea and vomiting are more likely to happen.

Risk of nausea and vomiting

Every cancer therapy has a risk of causing side effects. These side effects can happen before, during, or after treatment. Your doctor or care provider will select an antiemetic treatment based on your cancer therapy's risk of causing nausea and vomiting. The risk of these side effects depends on the specific treatment type and the part of your body that's being treated.

Sometimes cancer therapies are combined, which may increase the risk of side effects. If you're getting more than one cancer therapy, your health care providers will base your antiemesis plan on the cancer therapy with the highest risk of side effects. Your care team

Guide 3
Cancer drugs with moderate to high risk of nausea and vomiting

Oral drugs (pills, tablets, capsules)

Generic name	Brand name
avapritinib	Ayvakit
azacitidine	Onureg
binimetinib	Mektovi
bosutinib*	Bosulif
busulfan*	Busulfex
cabozantinib	Cabometyx
ceritinib	Zykadia
crizotinib	Xalkori
cyclophosphamide*	–
dabrafenib	Tafinlar
enasidenib	Idhifa
encorafenib	Braftovi
estramustine	Emcyt
etoposide	–
fedratinib	Inrebic
imatinib*	Gleevec
lenvatinib*	Lenvima
lomustine	Gleostine
midostaurin	Rydapt
mitotane	Lysodren
mobocertinib	Exkivity
niraparib	Zejula
olaparib	Lynparza
procarbazine	Matulane
rucaparib	Rubraca
selinexor	Xpovio
temozolomide*	Temodar

** higher dose version*

will also consider other factors that put you at risk for nausea and vomiting, such as those in Guide 1 (page 8).

Risks from chemotherapy drugs

Chemotherapy drugs are grouped into 4 levels based on their risk of causing nausea and vomiting: high, moderate, low, and minimal. The higher the drug's risk level, the more likely it is to cause nausea and vomiting.

When patients *don't* get antiemetic medication before high-risk chemotherapy, most have the side effect of vomiting. But when patients *do* get antiemetic treatment before high-risk chemotherapy, a lot fewer of them develop vomiting.

To assess the level of risk, your care team will also consider the form of cancer therapy. These therapies include drugs injected into your body (IVs and injections) and those you swallow (pills, tablets, and capsules).

Cancer drugs with moderate to high risk (including chemotherapies, immunotherapies, and targeted therapies) that are taken by swallowing are listed in Guide 3.

Cancer drugs with high risk (including chemotherapies, immunotherapies, and targeted therapies) that are given by IV or injection are listed in Guide 4.

Guide 4
Cancer drugs with high risk of nausea and vomiting

IV and injectable drugs

Generic name	Brand name
carboplatin	–
carmustine*	–
cisplatin	–
cyclophosphamide*	–
dacarbazine	–
doxorubicin*	Adriamycin
epirubicin*	Ellence
ifosfamide*	–
mechlorethamine	–
melphalan*	Evomela
sacituzumab govitecan-hziy	Trodelvy
streptozocin	Zanosar

** higher dose version*

Guide 5
Radiation therapy and risk of nausea and vomiting

Risk level	Area treated
High	• Whole body
Moderate	• Upper abdomen • Brain and spine
Low	• Head and neck • Chest • Pelvis
Minimal	• Arms and legs • Breasts

Risks from radiation therapy

Radiation therapy is more likely to cause nausea and vomiting when it's given in larger or more frequent doses, and when more areas of the body are treated.

Like chemotherapy, radiation therapy also has 4 risk levels. The level of risk is based on the areas of the body being given radiation. The highest risk for nausea and vomiting is radiation to the whole body. The lowest risk is radiation to the arms and legs. See Guide 5.

When chemotherapy and radiation are given together (chemoradiation therapy), the type, dose, and schedule of antiemetic drugs are based on the chemotherapy's risk of side effects.

Key points

- Nausea and vomiting are two of the most common side effects of cancer treatment.
- Sometimes the side effects of cancer treatment can be difficult to distinguish from the symptoms of the cancer itself.
- Higher amounts (doses) of chemotherapy or radiation therapy often cause more severe side effects.
- Your care team will select antiemetic treatment based on your cancer therapy's risk of causing nausea and vomiting.
- The types of chemotherapy-induced nausea and vomiting include acute, delayed, anticipatory, breakthrough, and refractory.
- The higher a chemotherapy drug's risk level, the more likely it will cause nausea and vomiting.
- Radiation therapy is more likely to cause nausea and vomiting when it's given in larger or more frequent doses, and when more areas of the body are treated.

Avoid becoming dehydrated. Drink small amounts of fluids throughout the day.

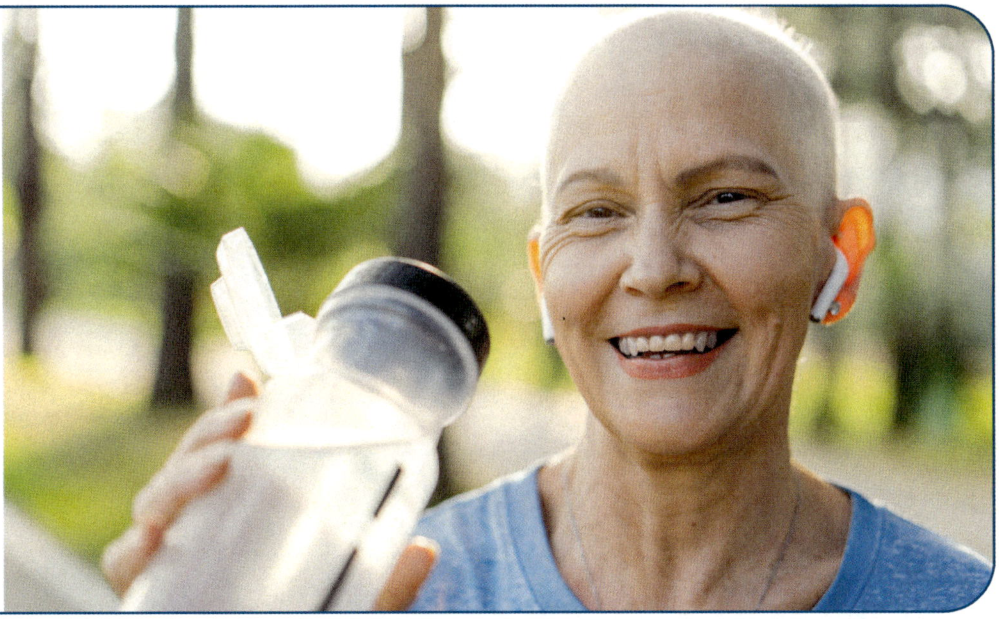

3 Preventing nausea and vomiting

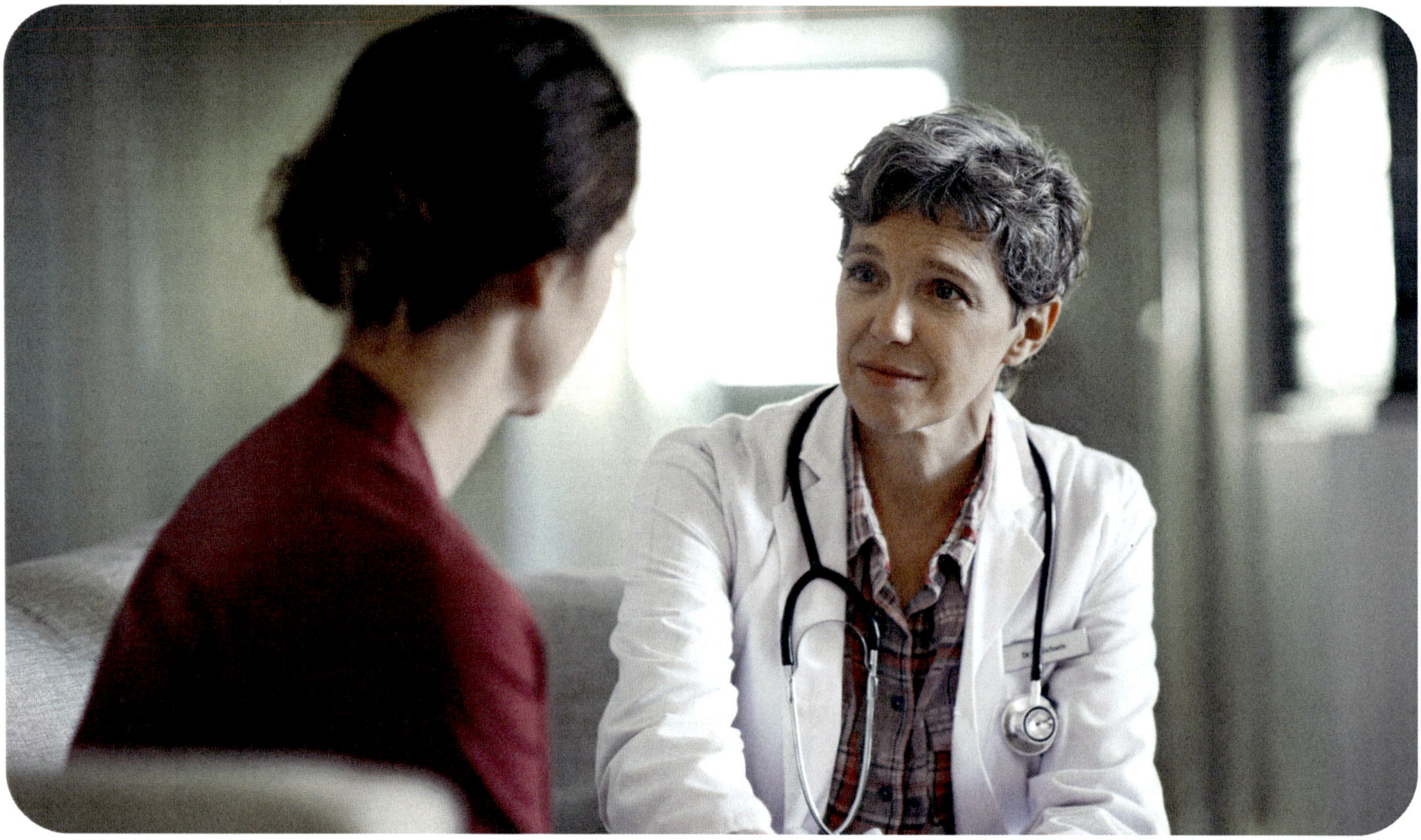

You and your doctor can make a prevention plan that may include different anti-nausea and antiemetic drugs. Continue to follow the prevention plan for as long as the risk of nausea and vomiting exists.

Drugs to prevent nausea and vomiting

Medication is the main treatment for nausea and vomiting. Most medications are taken before cancer treatment, although some can be taken afterward. It's usually much easier to prevent nausea and vomiting than it is to treat them once they've started. That's why this book emphasizes prevention.

Anti-nausea and anti-vomiting drugs are listed in Guide 6.

In addition to drugs, other types of therapy like meditation or breathing exercises may help you feel better. When and how much you eat can also affect nausea and vomiting. We'll discuss these non-drug methods in Chapter 4.

Doctors need to think about many things when deciding how to prevent nausea and vomiting. Your doctor and care team will look at the whole picture—from before your cancer treatment until after the last dose.

Things your doctor considers when planning to prevent nausea and vomiting include:

- Your type of cancer treatment
- Your level of risk for nausea and vomiting from the cancer treatment
- What anti-nausea or antiemetic drug (or drugs) to give you
- The side effects of the drug(s)
- The time to give it to you (for example, 24 hours before cancer treatment)
- How much you'll need (dose)
- Your past use of anti-nausea and anti-vomiting drugs

Timing of drugs

Preventing nausea and vomiting is the goal. So anti-nausea and anti-vomiting drugs are given before cancer treatment.

But antiemetics can also be given *after* starting cancer therapy if the therapy is likely to cause delayed nausea and vomiting. After the last dose of chemotherapy, the possibility that you'll start vomiting lasts for at least 3 days with high-risk chemotherapy drugs and 2 days with moderate-risk chemotherapy drugs. You should continue to take antiemetic medication for as long as the risk exists.

For cancer therapy with moderate to high risk of nausea and vomiting, your doctor can give you anti-nausea and antiemetic drugs on a planned schedule. For medications with low risk, your doctor may give you anti-nausea and antiemetic drugs only when needed.

The treatment may work better when taken at a certain time of the day. This might be in the morning or evening, once a day, or more than once a day.

If you have questions about how much or when to take any type of anti-nausea or antiemetic drugs, ask your doctor or pharmacist for more information.

Guide 6
Anti-nausea and anti-vomiting drugs

Type of drug	Generic name	Brand name	Forms available
Serotonin ($5\text{-}HT_3$) antagonists	dolasetron	Anzemet	tablet
	granisetron	Kytril	tablet, injection
		Sancuso	skin patch
		Sustol	injection
	ondansetron	Zofran	tablet, oral liquid, injection, dissolvable tablet
	palonosetron	Aloxi	injection
Neurokinin-1 (NK-1) antagonists	aprepitant emulsion	Cinvanti	IV push/infusion
	aprepitant	Emend	capsule, oral liquid
	fosaprepitant	Emend	injection
	netupitant/ palonosetron	Akynzeo	capsule
	fosnetupitant/ palonosetron	Akynzeo	injection
	rolapitant	Varubi	tablet
Atypical antipsychotic	olanzapine	Zyprexa	tablet
		Zyprexa Zydis	dissolvable tablet
Corticosteroid	dexamethasone	Decadron	tablet, injection
Benzodiazepine	lorazepam	Ativan	tablet, oral liquid, injection

(continued on next page)

Guide 6
Anti-nausea and anti-vomiting drugs *(continued)*

Type of drug	Generic name	Brand name	Forms available
Dopamine antagonists	prochlorperazine	Compazine	tablet, injection, suppository
	promethazine	Phenergan	tablet, oral liquid, suppository
	metoclopramide	Reglan	tablet, oral liquid, injection
	haloperidol	Haldol	tablet, oral liquid, injection
Cannabinoids	dronabinol	Marinol	capsule
		Syndros	oral liquid
Motion sickness medication	scopolamine	Transderm Scōp	skin patch

Forms of drugs

Antiemetic drugs come in different forms. These include the kind you swallow such as tablets, capsules, oral liquid, and those that dissolve in your mouth. Other antiemetics are injected into your body—into a vein, a muscle, or under your skin. Other forms are transdermal patches (placed on your skin) and rectal suppositories (inserted into the rectum).

Types of drugs

There are different types (classes) of antiemetics and even different ways they're given. Your doctor will recommend what's known to work for preventing or treating your type of nausea and vomiting. For example, scientists have found that 5-HT3 antagonists are the most effective type of drug for preventing radiation-induced nausea and vomiting. If you'll be receiving radiation therapy, your doctor may recommend a 5-HT3 antagonist with or without other medication.

The different classes of anti-nausea and antiemetic drugs include:

Serotonin (5-HT3) antagonists

Serotonin (also called 5-HT3) is a neurotransmitter that's triggered by cancer therapy to carry the vomiting impulse from the intestine to the brain. The 5-HT3 antagonists are a type of drug that blocks serotonin from reaching the brain, which can prevent nausea and vomiting. The 5-HT3 antagonists also sometimes decrease diarrhea, a troublesome result of radiation therapy.

The most common side effects of 5-HT3 antagonists are headache and constipation. Because 5-HT3 antagonists are less effective against delayed nausea and vomiting as they are against the acute type, they're often paired with neurokinin-1 (NK-1) antagonists and other medications.

Neurokinin-1 (NK-1) antagonists

NK-1 antagonists prevent both acute and delayed nausea and vomiting by blocking a neurotransmitter called Substance P. Substance P has dozens of functions as a neurotransmitter—one of which is setting off the vomiting reflex. NK-1 antagonists are drugs that prevent Substance P from attaching to the NK-1 receptors in the brain, which may stop or reduce the vomiting reflex. Common side effects of NK-1 antagonists include tiredness (fatigue), hiccups, and headache.

Atypical antipsychotic

Olanzapine is a drug that has been used historically for treating mental health conditions. But doctors have discovered it also prevents and treats acute, delayed, and refractory nausea and vomiting in patients receiving moderate- to high-risk chemotherapy. Olanzapine disables several neurotransmitters linked to nausea and vomiting caused by cancer therapy. It's typically given in combination with 2 or 3 other antiemetic drugs prior to chemotherapy, but may be given by itself or with other antiemetics after chemotherapy. Olanzapine sometimes causes drowsiness (sedation), fatigue, and dizziness. It should be used with caution in older patients and patients with dementia. Because this medication can cause sedation, it may be more effective if taken at bedtime. Check with your care team if you were prescribed olanzapine in combination with prochlorperazine or metoclopramide.

Corticosteroids

Corticosteroids (steroids) have been used for years to prevent both acute and delayed nausea and vomiting caused by cancer therapy. The main steroid used for nausea and vomiting is dexamethasone. If your chemotherapy already includes a steroid, you may not need dexamethasone as an antiemetic.

Steroids can have a lot of side effects, such as insomnia, upset stomach, and raised blood sugar levels. So the dose, frequency, and duration of using this medication are customized for each patient. Other techniques can also decrease steroids' side effects. For example, taking dexamethasone in the morning can help reduce insomnia. Also, taking dexamethasone with food can prevent an upset stomach.

Dopamine antagonists

Dopamine receptor antagonists were the first class of drugs used for nausea and vomiting due to cancer treatment. These drugs block the neurotransmitter dopamine from reaching the chemoreceptor trigger zone in the brain.

Dopamine antagonists can cause numerous side effects, such as sedation, dry mouth, constipation, uncontrollable muscle movements or tremors, and blurred vision. Older patients may be more affected by these side effects.

Cannabinoids

Cannabinoids are drugs that contain the active ingredient in cannabis (marijuana). Cannabinoids prevent nausea and vomiting by blocking receptors in the central nervous system's endocannabinoid system. The endocannabinoid system regulates many functions, some of which involve hunger and mood.

Cannabinoids are sometimes used to treat nausea and vomiting when standard antiemetic drugs haven't worked.

Cannabinoids can even stimulate appetite in people having cancer treatment. But they also have some undesirable side effects such as dizziness, sleepiness, lightheadedness, anxiety, mood changes, and other effects. Before using cannabinoids, ask your doctor about any possible side effects you might have.

Motion sickness medication

Motion sickness medication can be added to regular antiemetics if you have breakthrough nausea and vomiting. Because capsules or

Take your medication on time

It's important to take anti-nausea and antiemetic drugs at the scheduled time and dose, even if you don't feel nauseated. If you wait until you begin to feel sick, it may be too late for the drugs to provide relief.

Why did my doctor give me an antipsychotic drug?

For many years now, olanzapine (Zyprexa) has been widely used to prevent nausea and vomiting in people receiving cancer treatment. But olanzapine has been used even longer to treat depression, bipolar disorder, and schizophrenia. Scientists have found that olanzapine blocks some of the same neurotransmitters involved in both vomiting and mental health conditions.

Can I try cannabis?

You may hear that smoking marijuana or taking capsules, edibles, or drops made from the active compounds in cannabis (cannabinoids) will drastically reduce nausea or vomiting. You may hear that they'll dull your pain or help you sleep.

But before you take a trip to your nearest dispensary, discuss this with your doctor. And don't stop or skip your prescribed medications in place of non-prescribed cannabis products. The ingredients in these products can interfere with your current cancer therapy or your antiemetic treatment. Also, the active ingredients and effects can vary greatly between products.

One cannabinoid antiemetic medication (Marinol) is available and approved by the U.S. Food & Drug Administration (FDA). Check with your doctor or pharmacist to get trustworthy information on this topic.

pills may be difficult to keep down during breakthrough emesis, this medication comes as a patch applied to the skin behind your ear. The patch releases the medication through the skin and into the body. One patch works for about 3 days. Side effects include dizziness and disorientation (confusion).

Heartburn medication

Along with nausea and vomiting, cancer treatment can cause indigestion and heartburn. Drugs called histamine H2 antagonists (H2 blockers) and proton pump inhibitors reduce the stomach acid that causes heartburn. Brand name H2 blockers include Pepcid and Zantac. Common proton pump inhibitors are Prevacid, Prilosec, and Nexium.

Benzodiazepines

Benzodiazepines are anti-anxiety drugs. They reduce anticipatory nausea and vomiting by helping patients who feel anxious to feel calmer and more relaxed. Benzodiazepines are also sometimes used to reduce anxiety due to breakthrough nausea and vomiting. The main benzodiazepine drug for nausea and vomiting is lorazepam.

Benzodiazepines are used in combination with other antiemetic drugs. Their most common side effects are drowsiness, dizziness, and confusion. Benzodiazepines can also cause dangerously slow breathing in patients who are taking opioid-based pain medication. If you're taking lorazepam regularly, talk to your care team before you stop taking this medication to avoid unwanted side effects

Combinations of antiemetics

People who have cancer therapy that lasts for several days will need an antiemesis plan that prevents both acute and delayed nausea and vomiting. Antiemesis treatment generally includes more medications for the acute period (first day of cancer therapy) than for the delayed period (next 2 or 3 days of cancer therapy). But because acute and delayed emesis can overlap during cancer therapy, it can be difficult to come up with an antiemesis plan that's completely effective for every day.

Your antiemesis plan also depends on the risk of nausea and vomiting from your cancer therapy. Cancer therapy with a high risk of nausea and vomiting may require a combination of up to 3 or 4 antiemetic drugs. Cancer treatment with a moderate risk may include 2 or 3 antiemetics. Low-risk cancer therapy may involve only 1 antiemetic. Cancer therapy with a minimal risk may not require any anti-nausea or anti-vomiting drugs.

Remember that therapy that works for one patient may not work for another. So be sure to let your care team know if your anti-nausea and anti-vomiting drugs aren't helping. If the first drug or combination of drugs didn't work, your doctor can switch one drug for another or add a medication from a different class.

Radiation-induced nausea and vomiting

Some types of radiation therapy—to the upper abdomen or the whole body—may cause side effects of nausea and vomiting. Antiemetic treatment is given on each day of radiation therapy to prevent these side effects. The recommended treatment is a 5-HT3 antagonist (granisetron or ondansetron) with or without a steroid (dexamethasone).

When radiation is given together with chemotherapy (chemoradiation therapy), the antiemetic treatment plan is based on the chemotherapy rather than on the radiation.

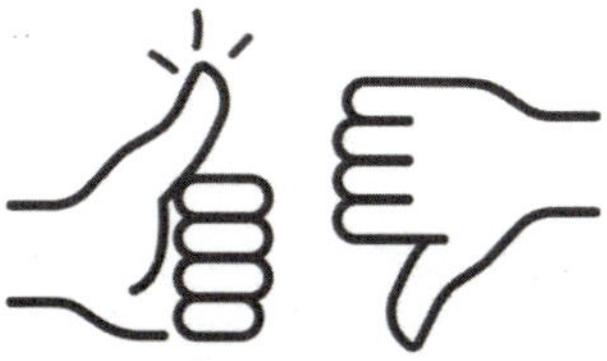

Let us know what you think!

Please take a moment to complete an online survey about the NCCN Guidelines for Patients.

NCCN.org/patients/response

Cannabinoids are sometimes used to treat nausea and vomiting when standard antiemetic drugs haven't worked. They also have some undesirable side effects such as dizziness, sleepiness, lightheadedness, anxiety, mood changes, and other effects. Talk to your doctor before using cannabinoids.

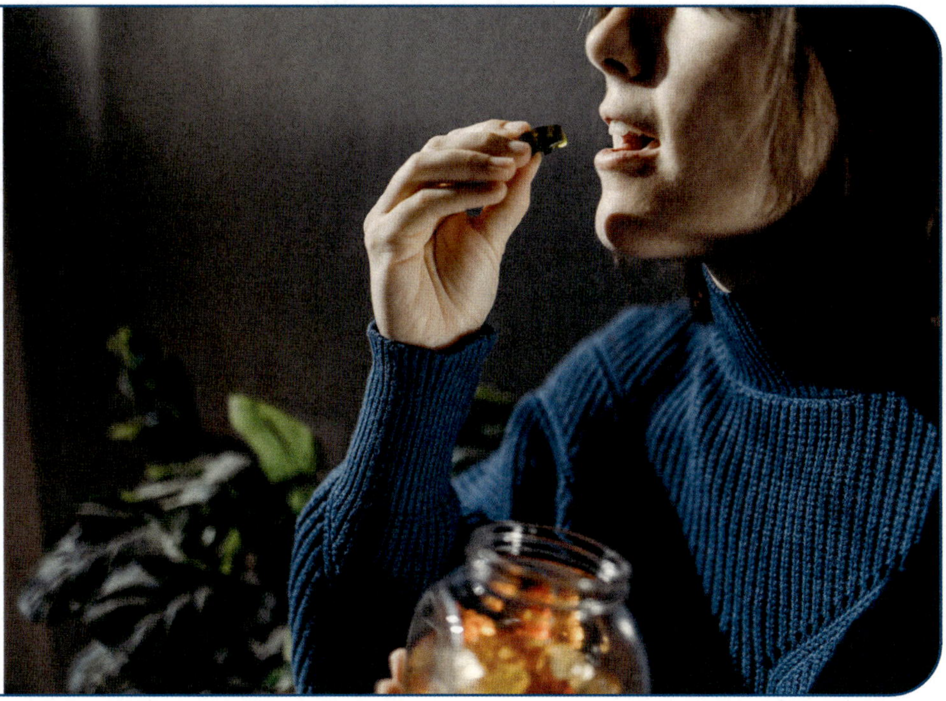

Key points

- To prevent nausea and vomiting, most medications are taken before cancer treatment. However, some are taken during or after cancer treatment.
- 5-HT3 antagonists block serotonin from reaching the brain, which can prevent acute nausea and vomiting.
- NK-1 antagonists prevent both acute and delayed nausea and vomiting.
- Olanzapine is used for acute, delayed, and refractory nausea and vomiting in patients receiving moderate- to high-risk chemotherapy.
- Benzodiazepines reduce anticipatory nausea and vomiting by helping patients who feel anxious to feel calmer and more relaxed.
- Cannabinoids are sometimes used to treat nausea and vomiting when standard antiemetic drugs haven't worked.
- H2 blockers and proton pump inhibitors reduce heartburn caused by cancer treatment.
- Cancer therapy that lasts for several days requires an antiemesis plan that prevents both acute and delayed nausea and vomiting.
- Antiemesis treatment generally includes more medications for the acute period than the delayed period.
- Cancer therapy with a moderate or high risk of nausea and vomiting may require a combination of 2 or more antiemetic drugs.
- Nausea and vomiting may happen when radiation is used to treat the upper abdomen or whole body.

Therapy that works for one patient may not work for another. Let your care team know if your antiemetics aren't helping. Your doctor can switch one drug for another or add a medication from a different class.

4
Managing nausea and vomiting

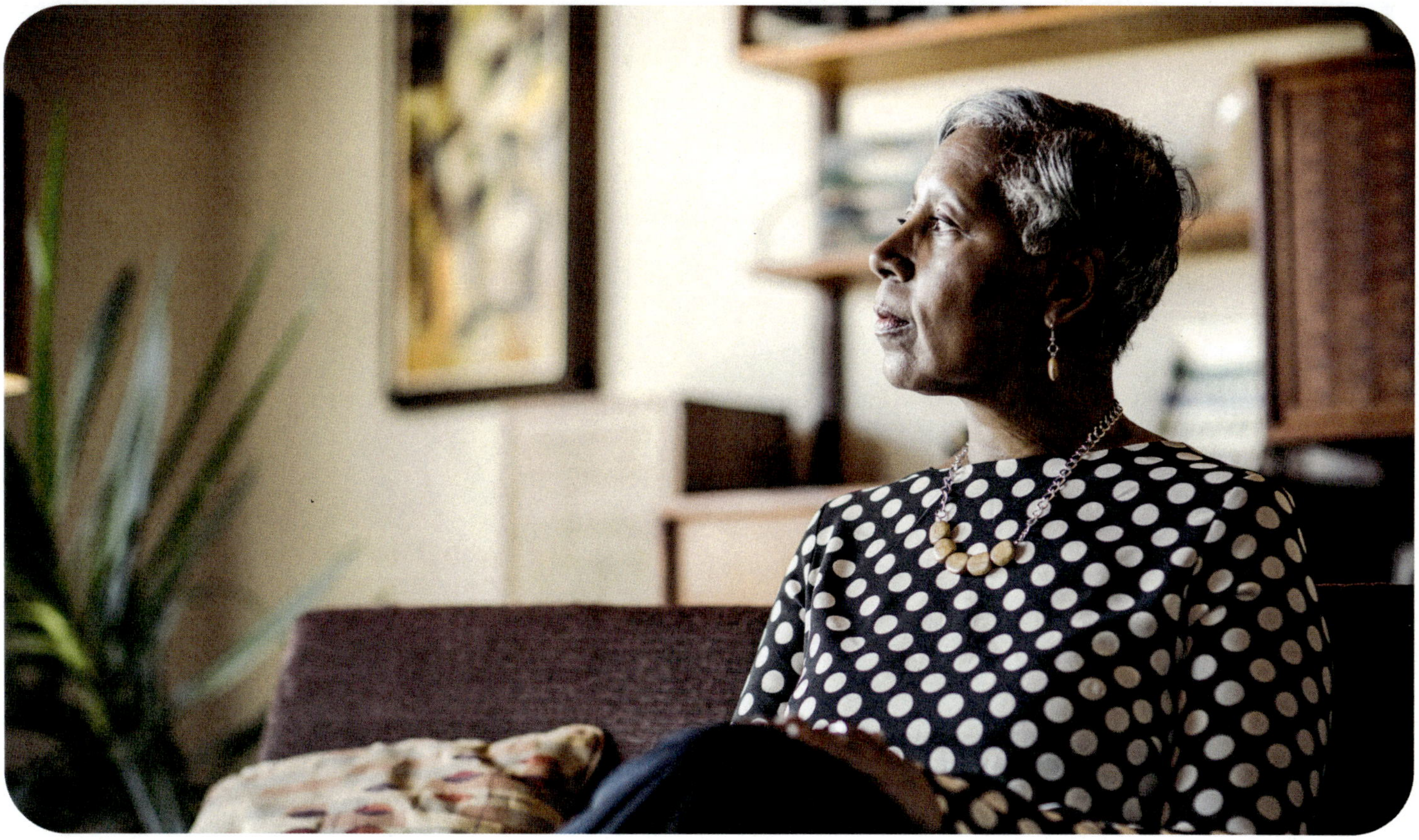

Even with prevention, nausea and vomiting sometimes happen anyway. This chapter explains various drug options and many non-drug strategies to manage and cope with these side effects.

Treatment if prevention doesn't work

Despite using antiemetic drugs before cancer therapy, some people still have nausea and vomiting during or after therapy (called breakthrough emesis). The treatment plan changes from preventing nausea and vomiting to reducing these side effects.

Your doctor or care team may ask you to try one or more of these treatment options for breakthrough nausea and vomiting:

Add another medication

The first option is to add another drug from a different drug class. The idea is to choose a drug that works differently than the anti-nausea or antiemetic drug(s) you're already taking.

Take several medications

You may need to take several antiemetic medications, each of which works in a separate way. This strategy attempts to block the emetic reaction at different points in the process. Your doctor or pharmacist may also recommend taking your medication on a different schedule or at different times of day. (Don't do this on your own without first asking your doctor or pharmacist.)

Go on an around-the-clock schedule

Instead of taking your anti-nausea or antiemetic drug(s) on an as-needed basis, you may be put on a schedule to take your medication around the clock.

Try a different route

If you can't keep down a pill because you're vomiting, you might be able to receive the medication in another form. For example, some pills also come as a tablet or a film that quickly dissolves under your tongue. Other methods include IV, injection, skin patch, or suppository (a medication placed in the anus). If one method gives you trouble, ask if you can try a different one.

See if it's something else

Before you receive your next round of cancer therapy, your doctor should check that there isn't another reason why you're having nausea and vomiting. Be open with your doctor about any side effects you have. There might be another cause that's related or even unrelated to your cancer. Other causes could be a lack of minerals in your body, stomach problems, or another disease.

Even something like heartburn can be confused with nausea. In this case, your doctor can give you antacid therapy to reduce stomach acid. Your care team may also help you find other ways to cope.

Keep track of your side effects

Your doctor may ask you to be aware of how you're feeling between visits. Pay close attention to when you're nauseated or when you vomit. You can write down that information and share it with your doctor. Your care team needs to know exactly what you're experiencing to be able to help.

Think about ways to keep track of your side effects. You can write them down in a weekly diary or create your own way to record any side effects you experience. Tracking your side effects in a journal or app may reveal a helpful pattern.

You also need to remember to take your anti-nausea and antiemetic drugs as prescribed. Use a calendar or an app to remind you when to take your medication. This will help you stay on schedule and, if needed, record any missed doses. Caregivers can also use these to help you take your medication on time.

You can try one of these smartphone apps to help you keep track of medications, appointments, and symptoms:

- Cancer.Net Mobile – A mobile app from the American Society of Clinical Oncology (ASCO) that allows users to track side effects. You can set reminders for medications and appointments, too.
- chemoWave – An app designed for people getting cancer treatment. It keeps track of your symptoms, medications, mood, activity, and sleep.
- Symple Symptom Tracker – A user-friendly app that allows you to track all kinds of symptoms, not just those from cancer treatment.

Report problems and ask questions

Your providers need to know if your antiemetic drugs aren't working. If the side effects continue or get worse with time, call your doctor or care team as soon as possible.

It's also a good idea to let your caregiver know if you're having any side effects. Your caregiver can help you track when side effects are happening, and knows what works best to make you feel better.

Another thing you can do in between visits is to make a list of questions you have. Review these questions with your doctor. Some people don't want to ask questions—perhaps they think their questions are unimportant or they're afraid of wasting the doctor's time. You need to know that your care team wants to help you by answering any questions you have.

Other people on your team can also answer your questions. Feel free to talk to your primary care doctor, nurse practitioner, medical oncologist, radiation oncologist, oncology nurse, pharmacist, physical therapist, psychologist, or social worker.

For a list of helpful questions to ask, see Chapter 5.

Coping with nausea and vomiting

In addition to treatment, several other strategies can help you cope with nausea and vomiting.

Eat small meals

Instead of three large meals (breakfast, lunch, and dinner), try several small, frequent meals throughout the day. Eating less but more often can be easier and less filling than eating fewer larger meals.

Drink plenty of fluids
Nausea can turn you off from eating and drinking, while vomiting can cause you to lose a lot of fluids. To avoid getting dehydrated, drink small amounts of fluids frequently throughout the day. In addition to water, electrolyte supplements (Pedialyte) and low-sugar sports drinks (Gatorade) can replace important minerals. Ginger ale or flat cola might help settle your stomach. Don't drink as much while you're eating, though—it'll make you feel fuller faster.

Eat to avoid more nausea
It's normal to want to skip eating when you feel nausea coming on. Surprisingly, an empty stomach can make nausea worse. If it's been a while since you've eaten, have a little food even if you're not hungry. As noted above, eat small portions frequently throughout the day.

Eat cool food
Hot food has a stronger smell and taste. If the smell or taste bothers you, eat food cold or at room temperature.

Avoid offensive smells
Common smells that never bothered you before may become unexpectedly unpleasant. Strong smells—or even mild ones—can make you feel nauseated. Smells you might want to avoid include:

- food while it's cooking
- scented candles
- hair products
- perfume
- smoke

Sniff good smells
Though many smells can trigger nausea, some smells have been known to help. For short-term relief, try taking long deep sniffs of a newly opened alcohol wipe. The smell of peppermint or sucking on peppermint candy may also "ease the quease."

Get some fresh air
A breath of fresh air can help. Breathe in deeply and exhale slowly.

Talk to a dietician
Ask your doctor or care team to put you in touch with a registered dietitian or a certified nutritionist. They can recommend ways to get enough nutrition even if you don't feel like eating.

Complementary therapies

Complementary therapies offer other ways to prevent or reduce nausea and vomiting. Complementary therapies are meant to be used alongside standard therapies. They shouldn't be used instead of your prescribed therapy. Talk to your doctor before using any type of complementary therapy.

Some types of complementary therapies used for nausea and vomiting are:

- **Acupuncture and acupressure** – These ancient practices use needles (acupuncture) or pressure (acupressure) to reduce nausea and pain. Bracelets for seasickness and motion sickness (Sea-Bands) are a popular form of acupressure.

- **Behavioral therapy** – A psychological treatment that helps change thinking patterns or behaviors.
- **Relaxation techniques** – Activities that reduce anxiety in the mind by lowering stress and tension in the body. Examples include breathing exercises, mindful meditation, and muscle relaxation.
- **Hypnotherapy** – A therapy guided by a trained specialist that uses hypnosis and the power of suggestion to relieve symptoms or affect behavior.

What to do after you vomit

This book is mostly about preventing nausea and vomiting. But what if you just threw up? Now what do you do?

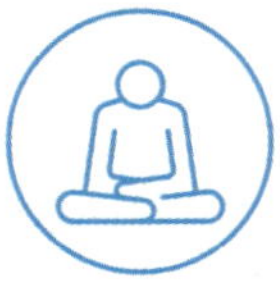

Sit and rest for 15 to 20 minutes. Let your stomach settle down before doing anything else.

Rinse your mouth. If you have a bad or acidic taste in your mouth, mix 1/4 teaspoon of baking soda into 1 cup of warm water. Baking soda neutralizes stomach acid. Swish it around your mouth and spit it out. Rinse with plain water.

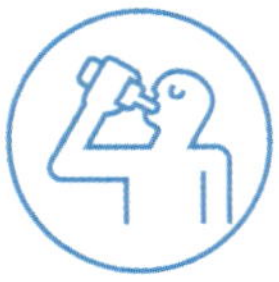

Drink slowly. If you've given your stomach time to settle and you haven't thrown up again, drink sips of water or suck on a few ice chips every few minutes. Gatorade, Pedialyte, and other clear fluids are good, too. After a while, you can try broth or Jell-O.

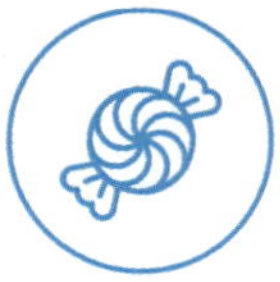

Suck on hard candy. Or lick a popsicle or a lollipop. These help produce saliva, which aids digestion and soothes your stomach.

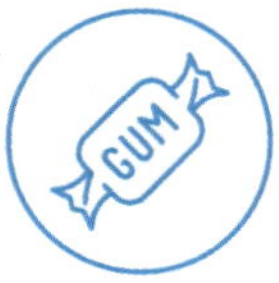

Chew gum. The action of chewing is believed to get your stomach and intestines back on track.

Try bland foods. If you feel like eating, and you can keep down water for several hours without throwing up, start with small bites of light, bland food. Try crackers, rice, toast, applesauce, or bananas. Go slowly. Avoid heavy, large meals and spicy, fatty, oily, or acidic foods.

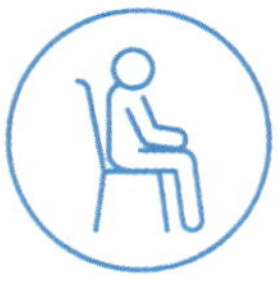

Sit up. Keep sitting upright for an hour or longer after eating. Lying down can cause indigestion.

If you throw up again after eating or drinking, start over by letting your stomach settle.

- **Guided imagery** – A relaxation technique in which a person visualizes positive mental images. This can reduce the anxiety associated with nausea and vomiting.
- **Music therapy** – A therapy given by a trained health care professional using music to encourage relaxation and enhance quality of life.
- **Ginger** – This root has been used for centuries to calm upset stomachs. Though more research needs to be done, some people find that ginger capsules, powdered ginger, or ginger-flavored foods and drinks (like ginger ale) help relieve nausea.

To learn more about complementary therapy, ask your care team. If you're interested, ask for a referral to a specialist who gives complementary therapy. Some cancer centers and hospitals have complementary care or integrative medicine programs for people with cancer.

You can also speak with a social worker, psychologist, or other mental health professional if you have any issues or need guidance.

Complementary therapy for anticipatory nausea and vomiting

Anticipatory nausea and vomiting occur in advance of the next cancer treatment. So prevention is important. In addition to anti-anxiety medication, complementary therapies can be useful, too. Some people find that behavioral therapy, hypnotherapy, or guided imagery can soothe the stress that leads to anticipatory nausea and vomiting.

Accept support

Taking good care of yourself is the most important thing you can do at this time. This might mean getting yourself healthier to prepare for treatment or staying on track with your treatment plan. It also means reaching out to the people in your life when you need help.

- Accept offers from friends or loved ones to do your grocery shopping or run errands.
- Ask a friend or family member to prepare a meal to help you avoid cooking smells.
- Ask your care team to help you find additional resources about nausea and vomiting.
- Be honest and let your doctor and your loved ones know when you're not feeling well.

Finding ways to cope can take time. Having the support of your family, friends, and care team can help you focus on the most important person right now—you.

Key points

- Tell your doctor if your antiemetic medication isn't working.
- Keep track of when you're nauseated and when you vomit. Share this with your care team.
- Remember to take your antiemetic drugs as prescribed. Use a calendar, ask a caregiver, or download an app to set a reminder.
- Eating frequent small meals may feel better than eating fewer large meals.
- An empty stomach can make nausea worse. Try to eat small portions throughout the day, even if you're not hungry.
- Stay hydrated by drinking small amounts of fluids throughout the day.
- Complementary therapies are sometimes used alongside standard therapies.
- Taking good care of yourself is the most important thing you can do at this time.
- Be sure to take your anti-nausea and anti-vomiting medication as prescribed.
- Many cancer centers and hospitals have complementary therapy programs.

An empty stomach can make nausea worse. Try to eat small portions throughout the day, even if you're not very hungry.

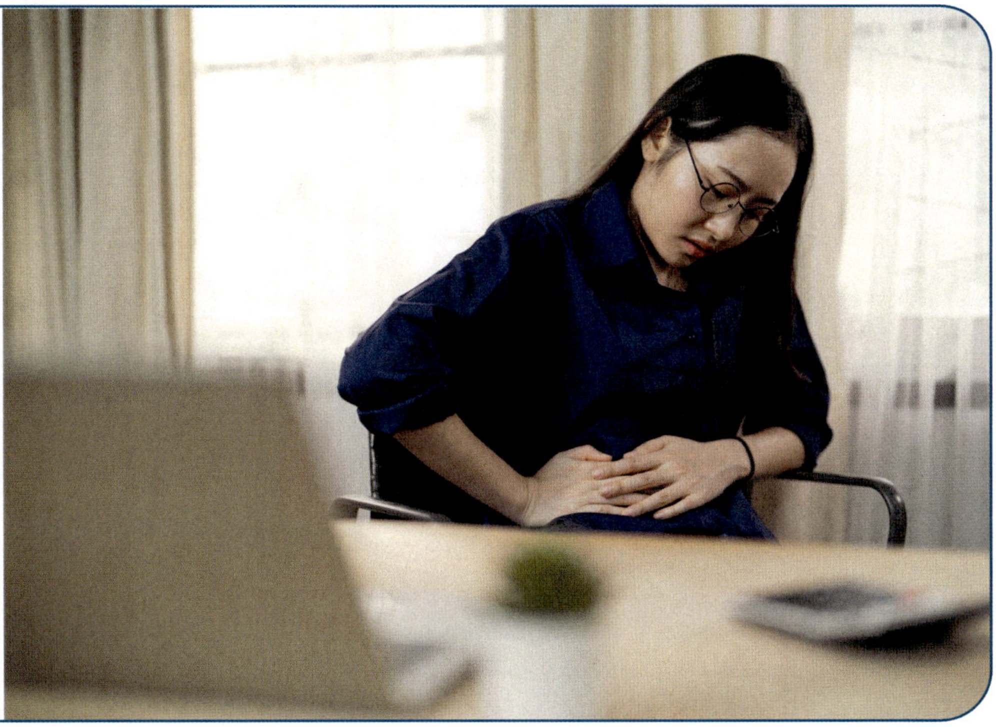

Report all your drugs and supplements

Let your care team and pharmacist know if you're taking (or want to take) complementary therapies like nutritional supplements, vitamins, or herbs. Some of these therapies can interfere with your cancer treatment or cause complications.

For instance, taking the over-the-counter supplement St. John's wort while being treated with the chemotherapy drug granisetron can increase the risk of a rare but serious condition called serotonin syndrome.

Put together a list of all the medications you take, including any herbals, supplements, and over-the-counter products. Make copies and provide this list whenever you have an appointment with a new doctor or specialist.

For more information on eating

Take a look at the National Cancer Institute's *Eating Hints: Before, During, and After Cancer Treatment* at www.cancer.gov/publications/patient-education/eating-hints.

Here you can learn more about eating small meals, having a full liquid diet, and avoiding foods that make you feel sick.

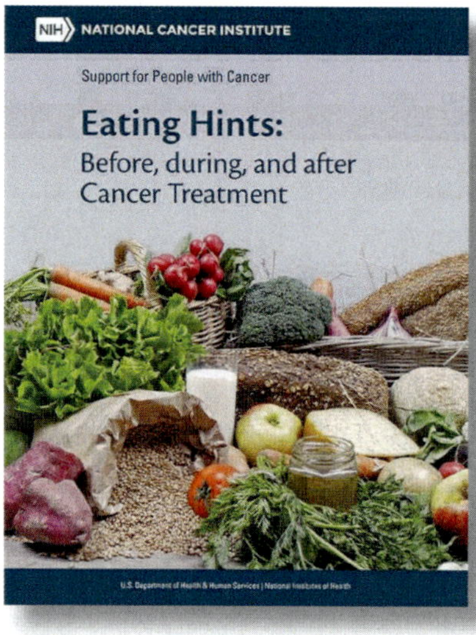

5
Making treatment decisions

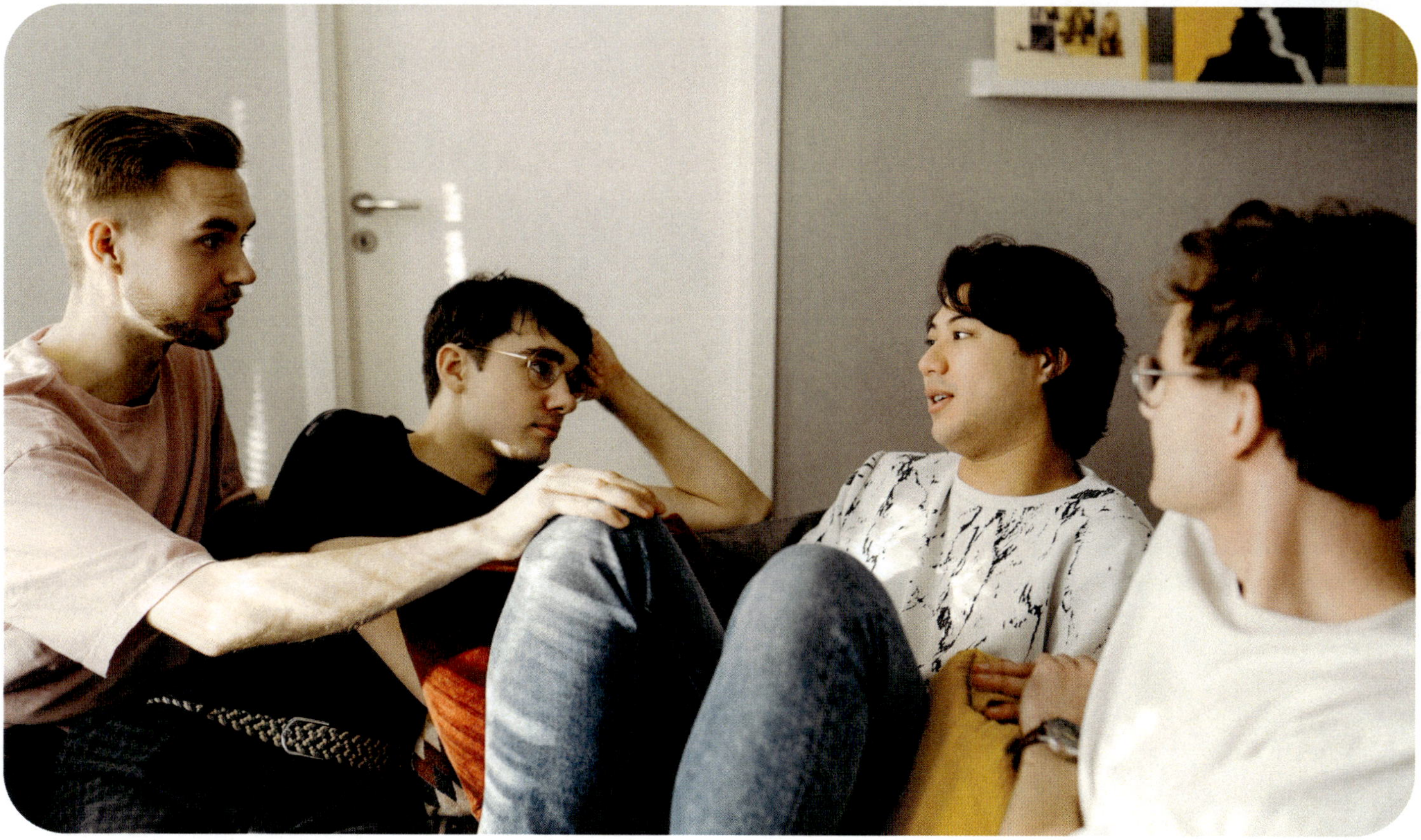

It's important to be comfortable with the cancer treatment you choose. This choice starts with having an open and honest conversation with your care team.

It's your choice

In shared decision-making, you and your doctors share information, discuss the options, and agree on a treatment plan. It starts with an open and honest conversation between you and your team.

Treatment decisions are very personal. What is important to you may not be important to someone else.

Some things that may play a role in your decision-making:

- What you want and how that might differ from what others want
- Your religious and spiritual beliefs
- Your feelings about certain treatments
- Your feelings about pain or side effects
- Cost of treatment, travel to treatment centers, and time away from school or work
- Quality of life and length of life
- How active you are and the activities that are important to you

Think about what you want from treatment. Discuss openly the risks and benefits of specific treatments and procedures. Weigh options and share concerns with your care team. If you get to know your care team and let them get to know you, you'll feel supported when considering options and making treatment decisions.

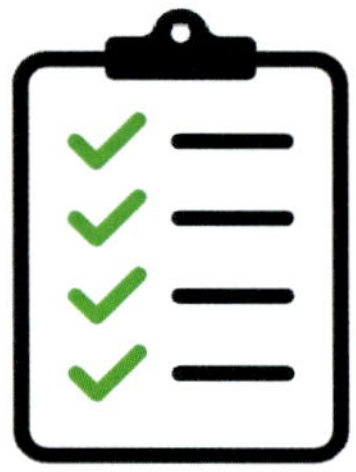

We want your feedback!

Our goal is to provide helpful and easy-to-understand information on cancer.

Take our survey to let us know what we got right and what we could do better:

NCCN.org/patients/feedback

Questions to ask

Possible questions to ask your cancer care team are listed on the following pages. Feel free to ask some of these questions or come up with your own. Be clear about your goals for treatment and find out what to expect from treatment.

Questions about side effects

1. What side effects can I expect from my cancer treatment?
2. When can they start?
3. How long will these side effects last?
4. Are there other side effects I should watch for?
5. Are there any long-term or permanent side effects?
6. Will you stop or change my cancer treatment if I have side effects?
7. What can I do to prevent or relieve side effects?
8. Do my age, sex, overall health, or other factors affect my options?
9. Do any medications worsen side effects?
10. What symptoms should I report right away, and who do I contact?

Questions about nausea and vomiting

1. Will my cancer treatment cause nausea and vomiting?

2. If so, when will it start? How long can it last?

3. Can I switch to a different cancer treatment if nausea and vomiting become really bad?

4. Could another medication that's not part of my cancer treatment be causing nausea and vomiting?

5. What medication can I take to reduce nausea and vomiting?

6. Can I take more than one antiemetic medication?

7. Does antiemetic medication cause any side effects?

8. Will my insurance cover the cost of antiemetic treatment?

9. What should I do if antiemetic medication doesn't work?

10. Is a clinical trial an option for me?

Questions about managing nausea and vomiting

1. What should I eat or drink to help with nausea and vomiting?
2. What should I *not* eat or drink to help with nausea and vomiting?
3. Can you help me find a registered dietitian or a certified nutritionist?
4. What other things can I do to prevent nausea and vomiting?
5. What if the nausea just won't go away?
6. Are there any complementary therapies that might help?
7. Will my insurance cover complementary therapies?
8. Do you know any specialists who provide complementary therapy?
9. Where can I find out more about preventing nausea and vomiting?

Resources

American Association for Cancer Research (AACR)
aacr.org

American Cancer Society (ACS)
cancer.org

Bag It
BagItCancer.org

CancerCare
cancercare.org

Cancer.Net
cancer.net

Cancer Hope Network
cancerhopenetwork.org

Cancer Support Community
cancersupportcommunity.org

The Leukemia & Lymphoma Society
LLS.org/PatientSupport

National Cancer Institute (NCI)
cancer.gov

National Coalition for Cancer Survivorship
canceradvocacy.org

PAN Foundation
panfoundation.org

Words to know

abdomen
The belly area between the chest and pelvis.

acute nausea and vomiting
Side effects that happen within a few minutes to a few hours after cancer therapy.

anticipatory nausea and vomiting
Side effects that occur in advance of the next treatment.

antiemesis
The prevention of nausea and vomiting.

antiemetic
A drug used to treat nausea and vomiting.

behavioral therapy
A psychological treatment that helps change thinking patterns or behaviors.

breakthrough nausea and vomiting
Side effects that happen despite trying to prevent them.

central nervous system
The brain and spinal cord.

chemoreceptor trigger zone
An area in the brain that receives emetic signals from the body and transmits them to the vomiting center.

chemotherapy
Drugs that stop the life cycle of cancer cells so the cells don't increase in number.

chemotherapy-induced nausea and vomiting
Nausea and vomiting brought on by chemotherapy.

complementary therapy
Treatment that's given alongside standard therapy.

dehydration
A condition where the body lacks enough water and other fluids to work normally.

delayed nausea and vomiting
Nausea and vomiting that occur more than 24 hours after treatment is given.

digestive system
A series of organs (including the stomach, intestines, and others) that breaks down food for the body to use as energy. Also called the gastrointestinal system.

electrolyte
An essential mineral in the body's fluids that helps control vital functions.

emesis
The physical action of expelling what's in the stomach out of the mouth. Also called vomiting.

esophagus
A tube-shaped organ that carries food between the throat and stomach.

guided imagery
A relaxation technique in which a person visualizes positive mental images to reduce stress and increase well-being.

hypnotherapy
A therapy that uses hypnosis and the power of suggestion to relieve symptoms or affect behavior.

immunotherapy
A drug treatment that uses a patient's own immune system to find and destroy cancer cells.

intestine
A long, tube-shaped organ of the digestive system that absorbs nutrients from food.

intravenous (IV)
A method of giving drugs by a needle or tube inserted into a vein.

long-term side effect
An unhealthy or unpleasant physical or emotional response to treatment that continues for months or years after treatment.

music therapy
A therapy using music to encourage relaxation and enhance quality of life.

nausea
The sensation when you feel like you're going to throw up.

neurotransmitter
A chemical messenger that neurons use to communicate with one another and with other cells.

quality of life
A person's overall satisfaction with their well-being and their ability to participate in regular activities.

radiation-induced nausea and vomiting
Nausea and vomiting brought on by radiation therapy.

radiation therapy
A treatment that uses high-energy rays (radiation) to kill cancer cells.

rectal suppository
A form of medication that's inserted into the rectum and absorbed by the body.

rectum
The last section of the large intestine ending at the anus.

refractory nausea and vomiting
Nausea and vomiting that keeps happening after each treatment cycle.

side effect
An unhealthy or unpleasant physical or emotional response to treatment.

systemic therapy
Treatment (such as chemotherapy) that affects the entire body.

targeted therapy
Treatment with drugs that target a specific or unique feature of cancer cells.

transdermal
Something absorbed through the skin.

treatment plan
A written course of action through cancer treatment and beyond.

vomiting
The physical action of expelling what's in the stomach out of the mouth. Also called emesis.

vomiting center
An area in the brain that controls the act of vomiting.

NCCN Contributors

This patient guide is based on the NCCN Clinical Practice Guidelines in Oncology (NCCN Guidelines®) for Antiemesis, Version 2.2022. It was adapted, reviewed, and published with help from the following people:

Dorothy A. Shead, MS
Senior Director
Patient Information Operations

John Murphy
Medical Writer

Laura Phillips
Graphic Artist

The NCCN Clinical Practice Guidelines in Oncology (NCCN Guidelines®) for Antiemesis, Version 2.2022 were developed by the following NCCN Panel Members:

David S. Ettinger, MD
The Sidney Kimmel Comprehensive Cancer Center at Johns Hopkins

*Michael J. Berger, PharmD
The Ohio State University Comprehensive Cancer Center - James Cancer Hospital and Solove Research Institute

Sidharth Anand, MD, MBA
UCLA Jonsson Comprehensive Cancer Center

Sally Barbour, PharmD
Duke Cancer Institute

Jason Bergsbaken, PharmD, MBA
University of Wisconsin Carbone Cancer Center

Caitlin Bowman, PharmD
Robert H. Lurie Comprehensive Cancer Center of Northwestern University

Debra Brandt, DO
Yale Cancer Center/Smilow Cancer Hospital

George E. Brown, RPh, MS
Case Comprehensive Cancer Center/ University Hospitals Seidman Cancer Center and Cleveland Clinic Taussig Cancer Institute

Jennie R. Crews, MD
Fred Hutchinson Cancer Center

Cassia Griswold, PharmD
Mayo Clinic Cancer Center

Christine Hong, PharmD, MBA
UT Southwestern Simmons Comprehensive Cancer Center

Andrea Iannucci, PharmD
UC Davis Comprehensive Cancer Center

Dwight D. Kloth, PharmD
Fox Chase Cancer Center

Kelsey Klute, MD
Fred & Pamela Buffett Cancer Center

Mark Kris, MD
Memorial Sloan Kettering Cancer Center

Dean Lim, MD
City of Hope National Medical Center

Cynthia X. Ma, MD, PhD
Siteman Cancer Center at Barnes-Jewish Hospital and Washington University School of Medicine

Renee K. McAlister, PharmD
Vanderbilt-Ingram Cancer Center

Rutika Mehta, MD, MPH
Moffitt Cancer Center

Lisle M. Nabell, MD
O'Neal Comprehensive Cancer Center at UAB

*Kim Noonan, DNP, ANP, RN
Dana-Farber/Brigham and Women's Cancer Center | Massachusetts General Hospital Cancer Center

Stacy Prelewicz, PharmD
Huntsman Cancer Institute at the University of Utah

Grazyna Riebandt, PharmD
Roswell Park Comprehensive Cancer Center

Jane E. Rogers, PharmD
The University of Texas MD Anderson Cancer Center

Hope S. Rugo, MD
UCSF Helen Diller Family Comprehensive Cancer Center

Ila Saunders, PharmD
UC San Diego Moores Cancer Center

Bridget Scullion, PharmD
Dana-Farber/Brigham and Women's Cancer Center | Massachusetts General Hospital Cancer Center

*Eve Segal, PharmD
Fred Hutchinson Cancer Center

Magdalena E. Seyer, PharmD
Stanford Cancer Institute

Maria Silveira, MD, MPH
University of Michigan Rogel Cancer Center

Suzanne Walker, PhD, CRNP
Abramson Cancer Center at the University of Pennsylvania

NCCN Staff

Lisa Hang, PhD

Beth McCullough, RN, BS

* Reviewed this patient guide. For disclosures, visit NCCN.org/disclosures.

NCCN Cancer Centers

Abramson Cancer Center
at the University of Pennsylvania
Philadelphia, Pennsylvania
800.789.7366 • pennmedicine.org/cancer

Case Comprehensive Cancer Center/
University Hospitals Seidman Cancer
Center and Cleveland Clinic Taussig
Cancer Institute
Cleveland, Ohio
800.641.2422 • UH Seidman Cancer Center
uhhospitals.org/services/cancer-services
866.223.8100 • CC Taussig Cancer Institute
my.clevelandclinic.org/departments/cancer
216.844.8797 • Case CCC
case.edu/cancer

City of Hope National Medical Center
Duarte, California
800.826.4673 • cityofhope.org

Dana-Farber/Brigham and Women's
Cancer Center | Massachusetts General
Hospital Cancer Center
Boston, Massachusetts
617.732.5500 • youhaveus.org
617.726.5130
massgeneral.org/cancer-center

Duke Cancer Institute
Durham, North Carolina
888.275.3853 • dukecancerinstitute.org

Fox Chase Cancer Center
Philadelphia, Pennsylvania
888.369.2427 • foxchase.org

Fred & Pamela Buffett Cancer Center
Omaha, Nebraska
402.559.5600 • unmc.edu/cancercenter

Fred Hutchinson Cancer Center
Seattle, Washington
206.667.5000 • fredhutch.org

Huntsman Cancer Institute
at the University of Utah
Salt Lake City, Utah
800.824.2073 • huntsmancancer.org

Indiana University
Melvin and Bren Simon
Comprehensive Cancer Center
Indianapolis, Indiana
888.600.4822 • www.cancer.iu.edu

Mayo Clinic Cancer Center
Phoenix/Scottsdale, Arizona
Jacksonville, Florida
Rochester, Minnesota
480.301.8000 • Arizona
904.953.0853 • Florida
507.538.3270 • Minnesota
mayoclinic.org/cancercenter

Memorial Sloan Kettering
Cancer Center
New York, New York
800.525.2225 • mskcc.org

Moffitt Cancer Center
Tampa, Florida
888.663.3488 • moffitt.org

O'Neal Comprehensive
Cancer Center at UAB
Birmingham, Alabama
800.822.0933 • uab.edu/onealcancercenter

Robert H. Lurie Comprehensive Cancer
Center of Northwestern University
Chicago, Illinois
866.587.4322 • cancer.northwestern.edu

Roswell Park Comprehensive
Cancer Center
Buffalo, New York
877.275.7724 • roswellpark.org

Siteman Cancer Center at Barnes-
Jewish Hospital and Washington
University School of Medicine
St. Louis, Missouri
800.600.3606 • siteman.wustl.edu

St. Jude Children's
Research Hospital/
The University of Tennessee
Health Science Center
Memphis, Tennessee
866.278.5833 • stjude.org
901.448.5500 • uthsc.edu

Stanford Cancer Institute
Stanford, California
877.668.7535 • cancer.stanford.edu

The Ohio State University
Comprehensive Cancer Center -
James Cancer Hospital and
Solove Research Institute
Columbus, Ohio
800.293.5066 • cancer.osu.edu

The Sidney Kimmel Comprehensive
Cancer Center at Johns Hopkins
Baltimore, Maryland
410.955.8964
www.hopkinskimmelcancercenter.org

The University of Texas
MD Anderson Cancer Center
Houston, Texas
844.269.5922 • mdanderson.org

UC Davis
Comprehensive Cancer Center
Sacramento, California
916.734.5959 • 800.770.9261
health.ucdavis.edu/cancer

UC San Diego Moores Cancer Center
La Jolla, California
858.822.6100 • cancer.ucsd.edu

UCLA Jonsson
Comprehensive Cancer Center
Los Angeles, California
310.825.5268 • cancer.ucla.edu

UCSF Helen Diller Family
Comprehensive Cancer Center
San Francisco, California
800.689.8273 • cancer.ucsf.edu

University of Colorado Cancer Center
Aurora, Colorado
720.848.0300 • coloradocancercenter.org

University of Michigan
Rogel Cancer Center
Ann Arbor, Michigan
800.865.1125 • rogelcancercenter.org

University of Wisconsin
Carbone Cancer Center
Madison, Wisconsin
608.265.1700 • uwhealth.org/cancer

UT Southwestern Simmons
Comprehensive Cancer Center
Dallas, Texas
214.648.3111 • utsouthwestern.edu/simmons

Vanderbilt-Ingram Cancer Center
Nashville, Tennessee
877.936.8422 • vicc.org

Yale Cancer Center/
Smilow Cancer Hospital
New Haven, Connecticut
855.4.SMILOW • yalecancercenter.org

Index

Made in the USA
Coppell, TX
18 February 2023

13000948R00031